"And Mr. Recorder, because thou art old, and through many abuses made feeble, therefore I give thee leave and license to go when thou wilt to my fountain, my conduit, and there to drink freely of the blood of my grape, for my conduit doth always run wine. Thus doing, thou shalt drive from thine heart and stomach all foul, gross, and hurtful humours. It will also lighten thine eyes, and will strengthen thy memory for the reception and keeping of all that the King's most noble Secretary teacheth."

Emmanuel speaking to Mr. Recorder
(AKA Mr. Conscience) in
The Holy War by John Bunyan

This book is dedicated to...

Zack De La Rocha

The Dalai Lama

Al Jourgensen

Jim Carrey

and Bono

The
John O'Sullivan
Diet
Fruit and Nuts

My Manifesto and
a Diet for Healing

John O'Sullivan

Published by
Pan Music Publishing

Copyright © 2022
by John O'Sullivan

First Edition

ISBN 978-1-8381219-8-3

Contents

Introduction

Chapter One of this book is My Manifesto which I first published as a free PDF on my website in May 2022 and updated regularly in the months that followed. Many people will be offended by it and much of it will be controversial but these are my beliefs and I want to share them.

The rest of the book is about a vegan, and ultimately fruitarian, diet which I believe will prevent, treat and often cure many, if not most, common illnesses.

I repeat myself many times in this book which will annoy some but bear with me.

My own approach to diet was inspired by three books which I highly recommend...

Fit For Life by Harvey and Marilyn Diamond

Raw Energy by Leslie and Susannah Kenton

Food Combining for Health by Doris Grant and Jean Joice

I was also inspired by the story of The Garden of Eden in The Bible.

I deem sunflower, pumpkin and sesame seeds to be acceptable eating as well even though technically they are not nuts.

Chapter One
My Manifesto

Part 1 (begun 7th May, 2022)

The first part of this article gives an account of my history of 'mental illness' and how I treated it by quitting drugs, cigarettes and beer and by embarking on a vegan, and ultimately fruitarian, diet.

Later parts of the article describe my views on the killing, and factory farming, of animals, treatment of disease through proper diet, electricity, the conflict between Muslims and Jews, the Mark of the Beast (666) in Revelation, Abortion, Jews and Judaism, Muslims and Islam, Zack de la Rocha and Rage Against the Machine and UFOs and alien abductions.

I was born on the 4th of March 1970. From as far back as I can remember I was never a lover of meat (flesh). Roast beef didn't do it for me. Roast chicken was OK and so were slices of cooked ham but if I didn't have them I didn't miss them. I didn't like fish either although fish fingers in bread crumbs were all right.

And like most children I didn't like vegetables either. And I had very little interest in fruit as well. As a young child my favourite meals were chips (french fries) and baked beans, or beans on toast. I loved custard and creamed rice. I also ate a lot of sweets (including chocolate) and enjoyed drinking cans of sugary cola. I was a fat kid growing up.

Shoot forward to around 1988 (I was around 18). Someone (a vegetarian friend of mine if I remember correctly) suggested that I go vegetarian. I thought about if for a while and it seemed like a natural choice. Meat never did it for me so the transition was easy.

I never looked back. I noticed after a week or two that I felt calmer, more peaceful, and I attributed this to going vegetarian.

Apart from a few rare occasions I never had any desire to eat meat again.

About two years later I was in college in Dublin and my roommate noticed that I intended to have bar of chocolate and a can of cola for breakfast. He told me that that was bad for my health. I had no idea! Some time later he gave me a book called Fit For Life by Harvey and Marilyn Diamond (this book was huge when it came out and was a best seller).

The book clearly delineated what foods were good for you and what foods were bad for you and why. Once I started reading the book I couldn't put it down. The enthusiasm of the authors was contagious. I couldn't wait to try the new regime they proposed.

The gist of the diet most people should be aware of by now... Eat lots of fruit and vegetables. Nuts, seeds, beans and grains are good. Flesh foods are to be avoided, and dairy products are not too hot either and should also be avoided, and we all know that refined sugar is a killer. (I've been on a strict vegan diet since around February 2021. At the time of writing it is the 6th of May, 2022. It's a bland diet but it definitely works, I'll be sticking to it.)

Unfortunately, no matter how eager I was to try the new diet I couldn't bring myself to make the necessary changes. I was still a vegetarian. Fruit still didn't appeal to me, neither did vegetables unless they were cooked in a quiche or a pizza. I think I may have cut down on my sugar intake but that was about it. There's a line from The Matrix, I think Morpheus said it: "There's a difference between knowing the path, and walking the path" I knew the path but I wasn't walking it.

Not long after this, 1990 I think, while still in college in Dublin, I took two tabs of LSD (acid) one night. This was one of the worst mistakes I ever made in my life. Too much of that stuff will melt your brain, it certainly melted mine. My personality changed overnight. My "mental illness" started that night and from 1996 until now I have been taking psychiatric medication. My advice to any young person reading this who is considering experimenting with LSD: don't touch it! You have been warned.

Four years later, in 1994, I had my first, and worst, nervous breakdown. I was bulimic at the time, and smoked cigarettes. I felt that I was damned by God and was going to hell and there was no way back, I was beyond redemption. I asked God why He had damned me. I flipped open my bible and this is the verse that I read...

Ezekiel 5:11
because thou hast defiled my sanctuary with all thy detestable things, and with all thine abominations, therefore will I also diminish thee; neither shall mine eye spare, neither will I have any pity.

To say I was scared would be an understatement. I was petrified. That was the 4th of March, 1994, my 24th birthday. I lived with fear, in varying degrees, from that day until the 20th March 2021 (27 years of fear). I have a good story about the day I conquered my fear.

I wasn't hospitalised or treated by a doctor until about two years after my breakdown. I moved out of home (I had been living with my parents) to a town 12 miles west: Clonakilty. I signed up for unemployment benefit. After a few months I decided to start giving guitar lessons (legally, I was on a Back to Work social welfare scheme).

Noel Redding (ex The Jimi Hendrix Experience) lived near Clonakilty and used to give me guitar lessons when I was around 15 or 16. He was a brilliant guitar teacher. He also gave me some great advice for life. One piece of advice he gave me was to never sign anything without reading it first. In 2002 I worked briefly as a computer programmer. I was given a contract to sign. Many people would not bother to read their work contracts but I read mine. There was a clause in my contract that said that if I invented anything, or patented an invention then the company I worked for would own the rights, 100%. I was only supposed to work there for a few months (I was studying computer science in college (C.I.T.) and this was a temporary work placement).

But the clause did not apply for the duration of my employment, it applied for the rest of my life! This was clearly unfair and I refused to sign the contract.

Anyway, going back to my giving guitar lessons (around the end of 1994), I taught adolescents in pretty much the same manner Noel taught me. I enjoyed the lessons and so did most of my students.

At one point, I think in 1995, out of nowhere, I started feeling unpleasant sensations in my body that were very annoying and extremely distracting. The best way I can describe them is that they felt like what I imagine nuclear radiation must feel like when one is exposed to it. I don't know where the sensations came from, perhaps little green men in UFOs, but I know this: they were real. I wasn't imagining them. I had to give my guitar lessons while enduring these maddening distractions and it wasn't easy.

In 1996 I started going to a night club in Cork city called Sir Henry's and I took ecstasy (the drug) a number of times, whenever I could get it. For some reason the unpleasant sensations disappeared while I was on the drug and my relief was immense.

I do not advocate the taking of ecstasy. I have a deep mistrust of synthetic drugs. But I don't know enough about it to shun it either. Before it was banned it used to be prescribed by marriage guidance counsellors to their clients IIRC.

Eventually the sensations (and the feeling that I was being watched all the time, that something was trying to control me) drove me into a mad rage. I remember shouting to myself....

I'M MAD AS HELL AND I'M NOT GOING TO TAKE IT ANYMORE!

NO MORE PUSSY FOOTING AROUND!

I CALL THE SHOTS!

And regrettably I shouted at my family as well. They didn't know what to do with me so they either phoned a doctor or the guards (Irish police) and I was arrested and taken to a secure ward in a mental hospital known as Kevin's 3.

Between 1996 and 2002 I was hospitalised 5 or 6 times.

I have fond memories of Kevin's 3. I met some very interesting characters (other patients) there and the nurses were very kind. In those days you could smoke freely in the ward and I enjoyed lying on my bed puffing my cigarettes.

My friends would visit me and I told them to bring in a few cans of beer with them. I would drink one or two cans with them in the visitors room. If the nurses knew about it they turned a blind eye.

The main treatment in those days was a drug called Largactil (AKA Thorazine). It seemed like everyone in the ward was prescribed it. It wasn't too unpleasant but it had a side effect whereby you couldn't tolerate direct sunlight and would have to stay in the shade.

One time I shouted at a doctor and I was forced to take monthly injections of a drug called Modecate, and later Depixol. I was on these for I guess around six months. These were the worst six months of my life, far worse than the sensations, far worse than the fear. Every time I stood up I wanted to lie down. Every time I lay down I wanted to stand up. I felt compelled to walk a mile or two every day (presumably the more I exercised the faster I could eliminate the drug from my system). I was always extremely tired and always compelled to move around. I had no rest, or peace, at all, for months on end! It was pure and utter endless torture and torment! In appearance I looked, and moved, like a zombie.

Halfway through this period I complained about the side effects of the Modecate and they changed the drug to Depixol. It seemed to me to be the exact same drug as Modecate but just with a different name.

Eventually, after an argument with my father about it, I stopped taking it.

In 1997 my brother suggested I go back to college, get a degree, get a job and get a life. I was up for it. I applied to take Computer Science in C.I.T as a mature student and I was accepted. I gave that course everything I had. In first year I never once missed a lecture, always did my homework and studied hard for my end of year exams. My exam results at the end of first year were excellent, my average mark was 80%. You only need 70% or higher to get First Class Honours. I was very proud of myself.

Second year was tougher and I only managed a 2.2 (which is an honour, not just a pass) but a member of the C.I.T. staff told me that out of the 80 students in my year I was eighth on the list in the order of merit. In other words I was in the top ten percent of my class.

Third year was much tougher and mentally I was struggling and as a result I failed a few exams and had to repeat the year. The repeat year was even more of a struggle. I just couldn't get it together.

I wrote earlier about my work placement as a computer programmer. On the fourth or fifth day it was clear to me that I just couldn't do the job no matter how hard I tried so I quit on the spot. I think my father thought it was a cop out and he was annoyed. Not surprisingly I was brought to a mental hospital, Saint Michael's this time, across from the Mercy Hospital in the Cork city.

I was extremely disturbed at the time, I couldn't look anyone in the eye. A verse from the Gospel of Matthew passed through my mind: "If thine eye offend thee, pluck it out, and cast it from thee: it is better for thee to enter into life with one eye, rather than having two eyes to be cast into hell fire" (Matthew 18:9)

Both of my eyes were offending me so I tried to gouge them both out. I remember forcing my forefingers into my eye sockets so that the tips of my fingers were directly behind each eye. Then I pushed as hard as I could. My eyes didn't pop out as I expected. My left eye was badly burst (from behind) like jamming your finger into a soft tomato and bursting it and I did some damage to my right eye as well but it was not as bad as my left eye. I remember it clearly.

A surgeon operated, my left eye could not be saved but my right eye was okay, thankfully. I never complain that I am blind in one eye, I am always grateful that I have one good eye. I would hate to go blind. To me it would be far worse than being deaf or a paraplegic.

That was around May 2002 and I wasn't hospitalised again for 20 years. I was prescribed an "atypical" antipsychotic (apparently the "typical" ones weren't working). It was called Clozaril or Clozapine (for some reason many if not all psychiatric medicines have two names). I found it to be quite benign compared to some other drugs I had been prescribed. It made me drowsy which wasn't too bad but I would drool a lot while I slept.

I was offered tablets to stop the drooling but I declined. My understanding was, and is, that the drooling was a mechanism to eliminate the toxins in the Clozapine from my body. Taking tablets to stop the drooling would only ensure that the toxins would build up in my body, making me even sicker.

I was living at home and things were fairly stable. I remember being at a party in 2003 and someone passed me a joint. I took a few puffs, began to feel paranoid after a while and I swore I would never smoke marijuana again. Some people have no problem with it but it definitely doesn't suit me.

9

Some time after that I promised myself that I would never take any recreational drugs, of any kind, while my parents were still alive, because I knew they would be devastated if I did and they found out about it. I have had no recreational drugs since then (2003).

By the way, at this stage in my life I have no desire to take any drugs, I prefer to be clear. Although I allow myself some red wine. It relaxes me and my thinking is fine when I drink it.

In 2006 I moved back to Clonakilty. I was on 350mg of Clozapine daily (since 2002). I was still smoking cigarettes and would go out for a few pints pretty much every night. I viewed this as therapy. By day I would work on my music theory, writing programs to test various conjectures I had about tuning theory. This work started in 1995. It took me 21 years (thousands of hours of research) to work out my new tuning system which I call Eagle 53. With this new tuning tuning some notes are a bit higher than usual and some are a bit lower and it has many advantages over the regular Western tuning: 12 Tone Equal Temperament. If you want to know more about it check out my website...

www.johnsmusic7.com

I still wasn't too happy though. I was concerned about my eternal destination. Would I go to heaven or hell? I thought probably the latter. And I had no peace of mind. I remember lying in bed one morning (in 2012) praying the Lord's Prayer. I got to the last line: "And deliver us from evil". I paraphrased that line and said over and over again: "Deliver me from evil. Deliver me from evil."

It wasn't long after I prayed those words that I was made aware of some verses from the Book of Romans in the New Testament. These were Romans 7:14-24. Here are the verses...

14 For we know that the law is spiritual: but I am carnal, sold under sin.
15 For that which I do I allow not: for what I would, that do I not; but what I hate, that do I.
16 If then I do that which I would not, I consent unto the law that it is good.
17 Now then it is no more I that do it, but sin that dwelleth in me.
18 For I know that in me (that is, in my flesh,) dwelleth no good thing: for to will is present with me; but how to perform that which is good I find not.
19 For the good that I would I do not: but the evil which I would not, that I do.
20 Now if I do that I would not, it is no more I that do it, but sin that dwelleth in me.
21 I find then a law, that, when I would do good, evil is present with me.
22 For I delight in the law of God after the inward man:
23 But I see another law in my members, warring against the law of my mind, and bringing me into captivity to the law of sin which is in my members.
24 O wretched man that I am! who shall deliver me from the body of this death?

Yes, as far as I was concerned this was a perfect description of the condition that I was in. So I decided to give Christianity a go. I sat at my desk and said a simple prayer: "Dear God, I want to be a Christian".

After a day or two I decided that smoking was definitely a sin and it would have to stop. So I quit there and then. I haven't smoked since and I never looked back. Once my mind was made up, that was it, I never craved a cigarette since.

This was the pivotal point in my career of mental illness, this is when the tide started to turn and I started on the long road to recovery.

The day I quit smoking was the 13th of October, 2012 or thereabouts. I started thinking about the story of the Garden of

Eden, all the fruit trees. And the first sin in the Bible was eating something you were not supposed to eat. It occurred to me that perhaps an all-fruit-diet was the diet intended by nature and perhaps eating anything other than fruit might be a sin as well.

So I decided to go on a fruit-only diet, for 40 days at least.

It was hard. I was eating lots of fruit but it didn't satisfy me. And I was hungry most of the time. I did notice however that I had no indigestion whatsoever. I usually had moderate indigestion daily and used to take antacids daily. I was craving more substantial food. I kept taking my medication though, more for my mother's sake than for my own, 350mg Clozapine daily.

I lasted 30 days which was pretty good going. After the 30 days I went to the diner across the street and I had a veggie burger and chips (french fries). Mmm, very nice. It was late in the evening and I decided to go for a pint. I used to drink stout (if you don't know what stout is it is a black beer with a creamy-white head).

Something very unusual happened. When I got my pint I couldn't drink it! It tasted revolting! It was like drinking bleach!

I thought it must have been a 'bad pint' so I ordered a pint of a different brand of stout. The same thing happened. I couldn't drink it.

I decided to try a pint of lager. This didn't taste quite as bad as the stout but I still couldn't drink it. It was disgusting to me. I tried another brand of lager. The same thing happened. I tried a bottle of cider, I couldn't drink it either, it tasted like smelly socks.
I can't remember whether or not I tried wine that night. I don't drink beer anymore but I do enjoy a few glasses of red wine.

I was annoyed. My favourite thing to do in those days was going to the pub and having a few pints, either alone or with friends. And now I found I couldn't have an alcoholic drink. It seems the fruit diet had highly sensitised my taste buds to the point where I found beer undrinkable.

By the way, at this time I realised why stout is black. When brewers brew beer (lager) they roast the barley to a golden or brown colour. With stout however they burn the barley, they cook it until it turns black. I remember the taste of stout at that time reminded me of black burnt toast.

I resumed my usual vegetarian diet. After a period of time, maybe a week, maybe a few weeks, I was able to tolerate beer again, just about. I quit the stout and stuck with the lager which I figured was healthier.

This was the winter of 2012. I began my Christian studies. I never quite believed that if I just believed in the cross of Christ, that Jesus' shed blood atoned for my sins, then I would be saved and would go to heaven. I don't buy it, it's far too easy. For me it has always been The Golden Rule: Do unto others as you would have them do unto you. And this is not as easy as it sounds. It can be very hard sometimes, I know.

I like Christians though, I've seen a lot of them on the Christian TV channels. In general they're the nicest people you could meet, regardless of whether what they believe is true or not.

Instead of studying the Bible I decided to read some of John Bunyan's books. John Bunyan (1628-1688) wrote The Pilgrim's Progress which was, for a few centuries, the best selling book in Britain second only to the Bible. There are two volumes: part 1 and part 2. The Pilgrim's Progress part 2 is so strange to me that I doubt Bunyan wrote it, I'm very suspicious of it.

The Pilgrim's Progress part 1 is, for me, the greatest work of Christian literature ever written. It is utterly enchanting (to me at least). I totally Identify with the main character: Christian. Christian is more like a soldier going to battle than a lamb going to the slaughter. I highly recommend it.

I had read The Pilgrim's Progress in the early 90's. Going back to 2012 or sometime afterwards I read Bunyan's Grace Abounding to the Chief of Sinners which documented his struggle and his feelings of being condemned which I could totally relate to. I also read The Heavenly Footman, which was good, but the book that made a huge impression on me was The Holy War.

There were a few lines in particular (in The Holy War) that caught my attention...

——And Mr. Recorder, because thou art old, and through many abuses made feeble, therefore I give thee leave and license to go when thou wilt to my fountain, my conduit, and there to drink freely of the blood of my grape, for my conduit doth always run wine. Thus doing, thou shalt drive from thine heart and stomach all foul, gross, and hurtful humours. It will also lighten thine eyes, and will strengthen thy memory for the reception and keeping of all that the King's most noble Secretary teacheth.——

I identified with the character of Mr. Recorder and took these lines to mean that *I* was free to drink red wine, whenever I wanted and as much as I wanted. Over the last few years I drank red wine pretty much every night. I did not drink by day. If I was working on my books (which was usually the case) I would not have my first drink until after 10PM or 11PM. Every time I drank a sip of wine I would wash it down with a drink of water. I enjoyed it but I knew when to stop, when I had had enough. And I never had a problem with it.

I recommend The Holy War as well.

But I was still far from happy. There was a time when I thought maybe if I started eating meat again it might 'fix' me. So for about a year I ate steaks, pork chops, roast (free range) chicken, roast beef, cooked ham, lamb chops. Did it make a difference in my physical or mental health? No. I noticed that my stools were a lot stinkier. I gave up eating meat again and did not miss it.

Still no joy, no peace of mind, although I was a lot better than I was before I started my Christian walk in 2012.

What else could I try? I noticed that I could go out on a Friday night and have a good few pints and feel OK the next day. But if I drank the same amount again the following (Saturday) night on Sunday I would be a mess. The beer had to go. So in January 2020 I quit drinking beer completely and drank red wine instead (which I had no problem with).

But I still wasn't happy. What could I do next? What wrong thing was I consuming that I could eliminate? Going vegan (plant based diet, no meat or dairy) was something I had considered for years but I never tried it as, like most people, I found it far too restrictive. But something had to give so I embarked on a vegan diet around February 2021. (I always thought that drinking cow's milk was a bit weird. Picture a man down on his hands and knees sucking milk directly from a cow's teat. There's something not quite right about that image.)

I noticed within the first few days of my new vegan regime that I had no indigestion and no bloating. Definitely good signs. Over time I noticed I began to smell better. When I went to the toilet the usual foul smell was replaced with a pleasant fragrance (I'm not joking). Another good sign. I was going to stick with it.

What did I eat? I usually had a fruit juice for breakfast (not freshly squeezed, it was from a carton). Sometimes I would have toast with a vegan spread and some regular jam or marmalade. I drank water with this. I went through a phase of eating vegan 'chicken dippers' which were made of pea protein instead of chicken. They were OK. I used to make a stew from lentils soaked overnight and passata (a tomato sauce), or a similar stew using butter beans from a can.

Some nights I made sandwiches from slices of white bread spread with vegan margarine and tahini (I love tahini), mustard, lettuce and either tomato or avocado. I liked these sandwiches a lot. Sometimes I had a banana sandwich with honey.

I ate lots of hummus and guacamole. Last thing at night, before I went to sleep I would eat a few handfuls of raw cashew nuts which I found quite satisfying. And I drank red wine.

It seems I was on the right track. Then at 2am 20th March 2021 something amazing happened. Two days before this I had promised myself not to drink a can of cider I had in my bedroom because there was sugar in it. Later on I had an argument with my mother and afterwards I felt like a drink to unwind. I decided to break my promise and drink the cider. I enjoyed it, no problem.

But that night I had a terrifying nightmare and woke up scared. Because of the nightmare I thought I had made a terrible mistake when I drank the can of cider. That day I was afraid even to eat let alone have a drink. I don't think I had any food at all that day (the 19th). Mum and Dad went to bed around midnight and I stayed up watching the Christian TV shows as I usually did at that time.

I was thirsty, I wanted a glass of water. A thought crossed my mind that drinking the glass of water would be idolatry. It would mean that I loved water more than I loved God. It seemed that I should not drink the glass of water but trust in God instead.

This was it! I said to myself: "You know, I am sick to death of this fucking bullshit. Are you telling me that if I drink a glass of water then I am going to hell? Oh yeah? Let's find out."

So I went into the kitchen and boldly poured a large glass of filtered water. I looked at the glass for two seconds, raised it to my lips and then quickly drained the contents in a few big gulps. Immediately this thought entered my head: "The unpardonable sin!".

"Oh yeah?" I said, "Fuck you, I don't care!"

I went back to the sitting room and a young preacher was pointing at me through the TV screen and it seemed to me he said: "The unpardonable sin!".

"Fuck you" I said, "I don't give a shit!"

At that very moment, the intense fear that I had lived with for 27 years was gone. Whatever spell was over me I broke it that night. I finally conquered my fear, I was finally free of it! This was not long (a few weeks) after I went vegan.

In the bible there is a sin called "the unpardonable sin" and whoever commits this sin is apparently lost forever.

There is a scene in Indiana Jones and The Last Crusade where Indiana has to choose a grail (cup) from a large selection and drink out of it. If he chooses the wrong cup he will die. In the film Indiana chooses a plain wooden cup, fills it with water and gulps the water down. He lived, he chose the right cup. That is exactly like my experience in the kitchen gulping my glass of water in the exact same way Harrison Ford gulped his cup of water in the film.

———

Shortly before or after this milestone in my life I started jogging (I had had zero exercise for 20 years or more) I jogged up and down my parents lawn which is 22 metres long. I jogged about 700 meters every evening for about six months, until the cold weather set in. This made a huge difference in my well-being. After a few weeks I had a spring back in my step. I felt like a man in my twenties again. I felt like a young man again. Every time I came in from my jog I felt exhilarated. This was the life!

I remember reading one of Bunyan's lines from The Holy War around this time...

——Nor must thou think always to live by sense, thou must live upon my Word.——

I took this to mean that carnal pleasures were to be avoided and it was time to study the Word (I assumed he was referring to the Bible). So that's exactly what I did. I read The New Testament from cover to cover and wrote a short book about it. The book is called...

Some Observations on the King James Bible

Here's the link if you want to read a free copy of the book...

www.johnsmusic7.com/sootkjb.pdf

The New Testament is hard to read. It doesn't read like, say, a modern novel. I found the book of Hebrews to be so obscure as to be gibberish, deliberate gibberish in my opinion. And the Book of Revelation is full of gibberish as well. I invite you to read my book (mentioned above), I give plenty examples of the nonsense verses I found and the many contradictions.

Back to the vegan diet. I'm very lazy when it comes to taking a shower. When I commenced the vegan diet in February 2021, after a while I noticed that I smelled better and didn't need to shower as often (another vindication of the diet). I would stick my nose under my shirt, have a sniff and if I thought I smelled OK I wouldn't have a shower that day. But I always knew when I needed a shower and when I did I would take one immediately.

In January 2022 (the 17th I think) I had my usual sniff and thought I smelled OK and was good for another day. Then I thought about it and realised I hadn't had a shower in two weeks! I went to my mother and I asked her to smell my arm pit and tell me if I had any noticeable BO (body odour). "A little bit" she said, "but not too bad" (or words to that effect).

This was something new. Before this I was showering more often. It occurred to me that I had finally, and unexpectedly, detoxed. That after ten months on my healthy vegan diet I had eliminated most of the toxins from my body. That was my reasoning. I had read about detoxing for over thirty years but now I felt like I knew what that word really means, because I had done it myself.

I must point out that I had a very sedentary lifestyle at that time. If I had been jogging every day I would have been showering a lot more often.

So it seems to me that I had detoxed, cleansed if you will, my body. I could clearly feel it! Great!

Although I was enjoying all the health benefits of a vegan diet I wasn't enjoying the actual food I was eating very much. It was OK but I wasn't over the moon about it.

Again I started thinking about an all fruit diet but this time I was confident that nuts (not peanuts which I don't like very much and are actually a legume), raw nuts in particular should be acceptable as well. They are tasty (to me at least) and you don't have to cook them to eat them. And if you want something heavier than fruit to eat nuts are quite satisfying (to me at least).

I could write at length about raw food versus cooked but I don't have the time right now. I recommend the book...

Raw Energy by Leslie and Susannah Kenton.

As far as I know humans are the only animals on the planet that cook their food. Cooking food denatures it, many vitamins, enzymes and other vital nutrients are destroyed by cooking. With raw food you get much more bang for your buck.

So a fruit and nut diet (all raw) ticks all the boxes for me.

What about protein you may ask? We don't need to eat protein to make protein in the body. Cows eat grass. Where do they get their protein? The human body can synthesise proteins from amino acids. A diet of varied fruit and nuts should provide all the essential amino acids the body needs to make the necessary proteins.

And what about Vitamin B12 which they say is found only in animal products? A friend of mine has been vegan for 27 years and doesn't take B12 supplements and he is quite healthy. Harvey Diamond suggests in Fit For Life that the whole Vitamin B12 deficiency thing is a myth. I suspect that he is right.

And while I'm at it did you know that there are several well-known vegan bodybuilders. Do an internet search on "vegan bodybuilders" and see for yourself.

Note that acid tasting fruits (e.g. lemons and grapefruits) do not combine well with carbohydrates (e.g. bananas) and nuts are better eaten on their own, not combined with other fruits. The nuts I like include: cashews, brazil nuts, pecans, walnuts and pine nuts.

On the 21st April, 2022 I decided to embark on a strict fruit and nut diet. I had a fair idea that I would go through what is called a "healing crisis". I thought that the fruit and nuts would raise me to, what will I call it?, a much higher level of energy. And that is exactly what happened. After a day or two the fruit I was eating tasted ambrosial: the food of the Gods. I remember munching on a banana thinking it was the most delicious food I had ever tasted. I felt charged with energy and alive.

On the 25th or 26th of April 2022 I performed a very daring feat which I cannot elaborate on here for discretion's sake. I knew at the time that I ran the risk of winding up back in a mental hospital and that is exactly what happened. The guards (Irish police) were called, it was suggested that I go to the hospital and I went voluntarily. It is now Sunday the 8th of May 2022 and I am (at this stage) an involuntary patient in the Acute Mental Health Unit at Cork University Hospital. And I'm not sure what my next move is.

To be continued…

Part 2 - begun 13th May 2022

I have done some shameful and despicable things in my lifetime. I'm not going to write about them here but they will come out into the light sooner or later. But just because I'm bad, it doesn't mean that you are good.

I think that killing animals is an abomination. And I think that eating their flesh is also an abomination. I often looked in the fridge in my parents house on a Saturday night and would see a raw joint of beef which would be cooked the next day. I always found the sight of the bloody raw flesh disturbing. It often reminded of a horror film I saw when I was ten or eleven years old: Zombie Flesh Eaters.

Do you eat flesh? If you had the choice between killing and butchering a cow or a pig (or even a meek little lamb) yourself and cooking and eating it, or eating a nice vegetarian pizza instead which would you choose? Many, if not most, people who eat flesh would definitely shy away from killing and butchering an animal themselves. They would choose the pizza. Yet they are quite happy to let others do the dirty deed (killing and butchering an animal) for them. Are you one of those people? If you are then you are a heartless hypocrite.

Flesh eating occurs in nature. Lions and tigers kill and eat grazing animals. So maybe this means flesh eating is okay for us humans too. Personally I doubt it. I have been vegan for 15 months. In that time I have found that I hardly ever experience indigestion. I used to experience bloating, both as a meat eater and as a vegetarian. I never suffer from bloating now. I no longer have foul body odour. When I go to the toilet there is no foul smell. I feel younger and healthier and my thinking is clear. Chew on that!

Here is something interesting. In Genesis 1:29-30 it says:
—29 And God said, Behold, I have given you every herb bearing seed, which is upon the face of all the earth, and every tree, in the which is the fruit of a tree yielding seed; to you it shall be for meat. 30 And to every beast of the earth, and to every fowl of the air,

and to every thing that creepeth upon the earth, wherein there is life, I have given every green herb for meat: and it was so.—

God changed the rules just after the flood of Noah (about 1,600 years after Creation) and declared flesh eating to be acceptable...

—Genesis 9:3: Every moving thing that liveth shall be meat for you; even as the green herb have I given you all things.—

So it seems that before the flood of Noah all of humankind and all land animals were vegan. There are a lot of things in the Bible I don't believe but these verses certainly caught my attention.

And what about dairy products? Milk, butter, cheese, cream, yoghurt. Consuming dairy products is far less offensive to me than eating flesh but for a long time (25 years or more) I often thought it was a bit unnatural. As I said earlier: picture a man down on his hands and knees sucking milk directly from a cow's teat. There's something not quite right about that image. For me it is bordering on the perverse.

And like I said, since I gave up flesh *and* dairy products I feel a hell of a lot better. As they used to say: "the proof of the pudding is in the eating".

So I advocate a vegan diet. I wrote earlier about the few days in April 2022 when I ate nothing but fresh fruit and raw nuts. That was a very interesting experience. I felt very energised.

————

Factory Farming

Read these few lines I copied from the peta.org website...

Force-Feeding
Birds raised for foie gras (pate) spend the first four weeks of their lives eating and growing, sometimes in semi-darkness. For the next four weeks, they are confined to cages and fed a high-protein,

high-starch diet that is designed to promote rapid growth. Force-feeding begins when the birds are between 8 and 10 weeks old. For 12 to 21 days, ducks and geese are subjected to gavage (force feeding)—every day, between 2 and 4 pounds of grain and fat are forced down the birds' throats by means of an auger in a feeding tube. The Washington Post reported that the tube "is pushed 5 inches down their throats, and more food than they want is gunned into their stomachs. If the mushy corn sticks ... a stick is sometimes used to force it down." The birds' livers, which become engorged from a carbohydrate-rich diet, can grow to be more than 10 times their normal size (a disease called "hepatic steatosis").

Gavage meaning: the administration of food or drugs by force.

I think by now most people are aware of factory farming. It is cruel. An animal version of the Jewish Holocaust comes to mind.

Chickens, ducks and geese are crammed into buildings, are often force fed and some are fed arsenic which makes them lay more eggs. They never see the sky or breathe fresh air, they have no room to move around and live in constant fear, torment and confusion.

Pigs are also factory farmed. They live in concrete pens and have no earth or straw to lie down on. Because of their living conditions they become aggressive and attack each other. When the pigs are very young vets cut off their tails because otherwise the pigs would bite each others tails.

I'm only scratching the surface here. Go to the peta.org website for all the gory details of the *very common* practice of factory farming.

And what about testing cosmetics and new (so-called) medicines on animals? And what about vivisection? (look it up if you don't know what it means). It's just plain wrong. And it seems no one gives a shit. Most people say "oh it's terrible!" And then they go shopping the next day and buy a factory farmed chicken (because it's much cheaper than a free range chicken) and cakes and biscuits and other products that contain factory farmed eggs. They never read the ingredients of the products they buy because they just don't care. If you are one of these people you are consuming pain and fear and misery. You really aren't doing yourself any favours, the money you save really isn't worth it.

When I learned about factory farming in my early twenties I diligently read the ingredients of every product I might potentially consume. If one ingredient just said "eggs" I knew these were factory farmed eggs and I wouldn't buy or eat the product. If the eggs were free range the manufacturers would be sure to state this in the ingredients: "free range eggs". I like the motto:"Happy eggs from happy hens". There's a lot to be said for that.

Certainly I slipped up a few times but I can truthfully say that at least 99% of the time (over the last 30 years) if a product contained factory farmed eggs I wouldn't eat it. 99% is a good score. I am very happy that there has been a little less suffering in the world because of my diligent abstinence from factory farmed eggs and chickens. Good karma. I like to believe in karma. And since I turned vegan my score is 100%.

———

The Prevention, Treatment and Cure of Disease

Of all the books I have read about natural healthy eating (usually leaning towards veganism and raw, uncooked food) pretty much every author has suggested that a healthy diet prevents, treats and sometimes cures many common diseases. Diseases such as arthritis, dementia, asthma, eczema, ulcerative colitis, fibromyalgia, myalgic encephalomyelitis, cancer, heart disease, multiple sclerosis, depression and even schizophrenia. I believe this 100% but almost all doctors will tell you that this is nonsense. They subscribe to the "a pill for every ill" philosophy. As if all of these diseases are a natural part of life and of ageing. I have heard some natural health authors describe most diseases as being unnatural, caused by bad diet. I totally believe this.

Sadly my experience has been that when I meet people with various ailments and I suggest some dietary changes they just don't want to know. They would rather live with their illness than give up the foods they love.

I am diagnosed with schizophrenia and until 20th March 2021 I lived with almost constant fear for 27 years. If someone had told me I could have peace of mind if I switched to a diet of nothing but soggy cardboard I would definitely choose the soggy cardboard. No two ways about it. My fear left me not long after I switched to a vegan diet.

But my experience has been that most people would prefer to live in ignorance than to change their diet.

Electricity

I have serious concerns about electricity. I remember encountering an electrical installation (if that's the right word) in the town park of the town where I grew up. I was perhaps nine years old. There was a metal contraption maybe six feet breadth, width and height. It was surrounded by a sturdy high wire fence and IIRC there were one or two DANGER signs around it. A powerful hum emanated from the thing. An incredibly powerful vibration was coursing through it. It seemed to be harnessing an incalculable amount of power (electricity). I supposed that the device was powering the whole town (which had a population of about 3,000 at the time IIRC).

It scared me. There was something very unnatural about it.

And I have had a few electric shocks in my lifetime. Exposure to domestic electricity for more than a few seconds could kill you.

I read somewhere once that the planet Earth is a sentient being, that it has awareness. Whether that is true or not I have no idea but it occurred to me that if it was true then the Earth must be in a lot of pain from all the electricity flowing through all the cities and towns on the surface of the planet. And of course if Skynet is real, or the Borg, or the Matrix, or the Machine that Zack de la Rocha rages against then it is electricity that powers them. If we could pull the plug, so to speak, we could render them powerless.

It occurred to me that if I was on a fresh fruit and raw nuts diet I would not need a refrigerator, or an oven, or a dishwasher. What about an electricity free house? Candles for light and a wood fire for heat. Maybe wash my clothes in cold water in a tub.

At this stage in my life I have very little interest in watching television or listening to the radio. I like to just sit and think. And write of course. The only electrical device I would miss would be my computer.

What about food for the winter? Some fruits can survive the winter. I'm thinking of appropriately stored apples. And dried fruits will keep good for a long time: raisins, dried apricots, dates, banana chips and more. And nuts will keep over the winter as well. What do squirrels do in Autumn? Gather and store nuts for the winter.

Have you seen the film Avatar? That's the kind of world I would like to live in: Pandora, before the humans arrived. Impractical maybe but these are my leanings. I would hate to live in a city. A small town where the countryside is only a few minutes walk away would suit me a lot better.

I feel sorry for underprivileged kids growing up in inner city ghettos, concrete jungles. Nature is such a beautiful thing, especially for a child. It is a terrible thing to live a life separated from it.

———

Muslims and Jews

In Genesis God promised Abraham and Sarah that they would have a son even though they were old and Sarah was well beyond the age of child-bearing. If I remember correctly nothing happened for a few years and Sarah grew impatient and told her husband, Abraham, to sleep with her Egyptian maid Hagar so that they might have an heir through her (Hagar). Abraham slept with Hagar and she bore him a son: Ishmael.

However, Ishmael was not the child promised by God. 13 years after Ishmael's birth Sarah conceived (by Abraham) and she bore a son: Isaac, the child promised by God.

Sarah saw Ishmael mocking Isaac and told Abraham to "cast out this bondwoman and her son: for the son of this bondwoman shall not be heir with my son, even with Isaac".

Abraham was grieved at this (evidently he loved Ishmael his son) but God told him to hearken to Sarah and early next morning Abraham gave Hagar some bread and a bottle of water and sent her and Ishmael away, into the wilderness. They nearly died in the wilderness for want of provisions. I always thought that this was a mean trick that Sarah and Abraham (and God) played on Hagar and Ishmael. God prophesied that both Ishmael and Isaac would raise up great nations (the Muslims and the Jews).

So Ishmael and Isaac were half brothers. The Jews are descended from Isaac. Muhammad and many Muslims are descended from Ishmael. So it seems the Jews and the Muslims share common blood, they are related, they are half brothers.

And yet many (but clearly not all) Muslims hate the Jews. It crossed my mind that the reason for this hatred might be the way Hagar and Ishmael were treated by Abraham, Sarah and the Jewish God, Jehovah. If the biblical account is true then I think the Jews owe the Muslims an apology for the way Hagar and Ishmael were treated. I think technically, back then, the firstborn (in this case Ishmael) should have received the inheritance but it was denied Ishmael and given to Isaac instead. Plenty cause for grievance here if you ask me.

I would suggest that the President and Prime Minister of Israel offer an apology to their Muslim half brothers for the way Hagar and Ishmael were treated. It couldn't hurt and it might help the cause for peace in the Middle East.

Part 3 - begun 15th May, 2022

The Mark of the Beast: 666

Revelation Chapter 13

16 And he causeth all, both small and great, rich and poor, free and bond, to receive a mark in their right hand, or in their foreheads:

17 And that no man might buy or sell, save he that had the mark, or the name of the beast, or the number of his name.

18 Here is wisdom. Let him that hath understanding count the number of the beast: for it is the number of a man; and his number is Six hundred threescore and six.

For me these three verses were, for a long time, the most significant in the book of Revelation. Did you know that there are three sixes encoded in most barcodes? Here's how it works...

When you buy a product in a supermarket, or a book in a bookshop, there will be a barcode printed on the packaging or on the back cover of the book. The barcodes are composed of vertical lines. Some lines are thin, some are thick and some are in between. Also some lines are very close together and some are far apart. The scanner at the checkout desk reads these lines and translates them into numbers. The first and second lines correspond to a single digit number. The third and fourth lines correspond to a single digit number. The fifth and sixth lines... and so on. Every pair of lines correspond to a number. I see on the barcode on one of my published books that a pair of lines consisting of a thick line and a medium thickness line, close together, corresponds to the number 7. The corresponding numbers are printed below each pair of lines except for the first two lines, the middle two lines and the last two lines. These three pairs of lines are slightly longer than the others and no numbers are printed below them. These pairs are always two thin lines close together and, as I said, no numbers are printed below them.

What number corresponds to two thin lines close together? Sometimes a different encoding is used on the left half of a barcode but on the right half of a barcode a pair of thin lines close together *always* corresponds to a six (6). On the particular barcode I mentioned above, A thin line and a very thick line close together (on the left half of the barcode) also corresponds to a six, a different encoding to the right half of the barcode.

So, if we use the right hand side encoding, then the left-most pair of lines, the pair of lines in the middle and the right-most pair of lines correspond to sixes. In other words: 666.

A cashless society is not a new concept. I have read that it is possible to have *invisible* (to the eye but not to a scanner) tattoos of barcodes on the backs of our hands. When shopping, to pay we just pass our hands over the barcode scanner and the appropriate amount will be automatically deducted from our bank accounts.

I can see this being implemented in my lifetime. If we are all compelled to have a 'mark' on our right hands or foreheads, and we can't buy or sell without it, and this 'mark' turns out to be a barcode then it looks to me like this is the mark of the beast which the bible tells us not to take.

Revelation Chapter 14

9 And the third angel followed them, saying with a loud voice, If any man worship the beast and his image, and receive his mark in

his forehead, or in his hand,

10 The same shall drink of the wine of the wrath of God, which is poured out without mixture into the cup of his indignation; and he shall be tormented with fire and brimstone in the presence of the holy angels, and in the presence of the Lamb:

11 And the smoke of their torment ascendeth up for ever and ever: and they have no rest day nor night, who worship the beast and his image, and whosoever receiveth the mark of his name.

If I am going to be compelled to have a 'mark' on my right hand or forehead so that I can't buy or sell without it I think I will probably refuse it. I'm not afraid of it any more.

Abortion

My opinion on abortion is that it is murder with two possible exceptions. For me, the instant when the sperm enters the ovum you have a human being. Not a small number of insentient cells, a human being. If a girl or a woman goes to a nightclub and gets drunk or high, and takes a man home and willingly has sex with him and conceives a child then she is responsible for that child. If she has an abortion then in my book that is murder. If she doesn't want the child I suggest going through with the pregnancy and then putting the baby up for adoption when it is born.

The first possible exception is when a woman is raped. I'm not God and I don't know for sure but I think that if any girl or woman is raped they should have the right to an abortion.

If I was a woman and I was raped, and conceived, would I have an abortion? I don't know.

The second possible exception is where there is a threat to the mother's life. Here is a quote from Wikipedia about Savita Halappanavar...

—On 21 October 2012, Savita Halappanavar, then 17 weeks pregnant, was examined at University Hospital Galway after complaining of back pain, but was soon discharged without a diagnosis. She returned to the hospital later that day, this time complaining of lower pressure, a sensation she described as feeling "something coming down," and a subsequent examination found that the gestational sac was protruding from her body. She was admitted to hospital, as it was determined that miscarriage was unavoidable, and several hours later, just after midnight on 22 October, her water broke but did not expel the foetus. The following day, on 23 October, Halappanavar discussed abortion with her consulting physician but her request was promptly refused, as Irish law at that time forbade abortion if a foetal heartbeat was still present.[8]:?33?[10] Afterwards, Halappanavar developed sepsis and, despite doctors' efforts to treat her, had a cardiac arrest at 1:09 AM on 28 October, at the age of 31, and died.—

Maybe I missed something, maybe there is a third exception. I'll update this article if I come across one.

And don't think that the morning-after pill is OK either. Conception can occur within minutes of having sex. Here's a quote from verywellfamily.com…

—We know that sex leads to pregnancy, but how soon after sex could you really get pregnant? The answer isn't exact. It's actually a range—it could be within minutes or could take a few days.—

So if you conceive within a few minutes and later take the morning after pill then that is an abortion, and in my book, murder.

I had a vasectomy around ten years ago but even that isn't fool proof. The doctor who performed the operation either told me, or gave me literature that said: it very rarely happens (perhaps 1 in 10,000 cases) but sometimes a vasectomy somehow reverses (or 'heals' might be a better word) itself and the man becomes fertile again. I won't take that 1 in 10,000 chance now.

Even coitus interruptus (withdrawing before ejaculation) isn't 100% safe. There may be a tiny amount of live sperm on the tip of the penis that is expelled along with urine. And I won't take that chance.

And several times I have had sex using a condom and the condom burst. So condoms aren't safe either.

And the rhythm method (not having sex for a few days before and after ovulation) isn't reliable either as unpredictable ovulations may occur.

What about female sterilisation? Look at these lines from Wikipedia…

__Tubal ligation (commonly known as having one's "tubes tied") is a surgical procedure for female sterilization in which the fallopian tubes are permanently blocked, clipped or removed. This prevents the fertilization of eggs by sperm and thus the implantation of a fertilized egg.

While both hysterectomy (the removal of the uterus) or bilateral oophorectomy (the removal of both ovaries) can also accomplish this goal, these surgeries carry generally greater health risks than tubal ligation procedures.

Most methods of female sterilization are approximately 99% effective or greater in preventing pregnancy. These rates are roughly equivalent to the effectiveness of long-acting reversible contraceptives such as intrauterine devices and contraceptive implants, and slightly less effective than permanent male sterilization through vasectomy.__

And I found this quote on the net…

—Tubal ligation is an extremely reliable way to prevent pregnancy. Fewer than 1 out of 100 women will get pregnant within a year of surgery—

99% isn't good enough for me. I won't take that chance. And the oral contraceptive pill isn't 100% safe either.

I read somewhere that sex is for reproduction, not for fun. I don't intend to have any sex until I want to father a child.

So if you don't want to have a child I suggest that you don't have sex.

Jews and Judaism

I like Jews. Have you seen the film Fiddler on the Roof? That seems to me to be a good depiction of what Jews are like. In general they seem like good honest decent people. And a lot of them have a great sense of humour. Some Jews look down upon gentiles (non Jews), even hate them, but the way they have been treated by the gentiles over the last 2,000 years who could blame them?

I like the way Jews look and I like the way they talk. Some of my favourite musicians and actors are/were Jews. Lou Reed, Leonard Cohen, Mel Brooks, Woody Allen, Gene Wilder, Barbra Streisand, Topol, Alan Arkin (who played Yossarian in Catch-22). Albert Einstein was a Jew. I found Benjamin Netanyahu to be a very impressive and likeable man. And the most famous Jew of all was Jesus Christ.

But there are things about Judaism that I don't like. First of all I have heard some disturbing things about ultra-orthodox Jews. I have heard that the wives of ultra-orthodox Jews have to shave their heads and wear wigs instead. I have heard that when ultra-orthodox jewish husbands and wives have sex their bodies are separated by a sheet that has a hole in it through which their genitalia meet. Someone please tell me that these aren't true, that these are lies concocted by anti-semites to defame the Jews.

Regular faithful Jews (not fanatical) are fine in my book, as are secular (non religious) Jews. But I have a big problem with The Torah (The Law), the first five books of the Old Testament. The problem I have is with animal sacrifice. The idea that killing cows, bulls, sheep, goats, and birds and possibly other animals atones for, or covers, sin is nonsense to me. That the shedding of blood atones for sin. I just don't buy it. And while I'm at it I don't believe that Jesus's shed blood atoned for my sins either (if I just believe it). For me it's what Jesus said that counts, not his blood. He said:"Do unto others as you would have them do unto you". For me His blood is irrelevant.

It seems to be very fashionable nowadays to hate the Jews. From watching various programmes and news shows on Christian TV channels (e.g. Jerusalem Dateline and The Middle East Report) I learned that the Western media news programmes are deliberately distorting the truth about conflicts in Israel and Gaza. The Jews are always portrayed as the aggressors, the bad guys, when the truth is the exact opposite. And all the Jew-haters lap up these lies greedily and feel that they are 'righteous' because they hate the Jews.

Israel is not an apartheid state. Muslims can vote or run for office. There are Muslim politicians in the Knesset. Muslims can share public transport with Jews. Officially Muslim Israelis have the exact same rights as Jewish Israelis. Unfortunately there are militant muslim extremists living in Israel and the Jews, naturally, have to protect themselves from these so some Muslim areas are cordoned off. IIRC working Muslims in Israel earn much more than they would if they lived in one of the neighbouring Muslim countries and many of them secretly (they would be punished by their peers if they openly said it) prefer to live in Israel. Many muslims have no problems with Jews but again they are afraid to come out and say it publicly.

If you are a Christian you should know that God promised that because of their sin the Jews would be scattered across the four corners of the Earth (which began in 70AD) but that in the last days He would restore them to the land of Israel. So don't blame the Jews for "occupying" Israel, blame God!

I am pro Israel and pro Jew. Israel is a democratic state. I would much rather live under a Jewish government than a Muslim government. Many if not most of the countries known for severe human rights abuses are Muslim countries (e.g. Iran).

———————

Muslims and Islam

I would love to read The Koran and write an article about it but I don't have the time. Any non Muslim is known as an infidel. Here are two verses from the Koran about infidels…

Surah 9:123 Believers! Fight against the unbelievers who live around you; and let them find in you sternness. Know that Allah is with the God-fearing.

Surah 66:9 O you Prophet, strive with the steadfast disbelievers, and the hypocrites, and be harsh with them; and their abode will be Hell; and miserable is the Destiny!

Many if not most Muslims (in Muslim countries) live in fear. If they do or say anything that could be construed as blasphemy (e.g. "I don't believe in Muhammad" or "I want to be a Christian") they will likely be arrested, imprisoned, usually tortured and possibly executed.

I am sure that many Muslims are very nice people. And I am sure that many Muslims would rather not be Muslims. But to speak openly about this would be suicide. They have to keep up the charade, pretending to be devout Muslims when in reality they are being oppressed.

There is a lot of evil in the world perpetrated in the name of Allah. These terrorist groups come to mind: Boko Haram, Hezbollah, Hamas, The Taliban, Isis, Al Qaeda (the latter responsible for the 9/11 attacks). I have heard of some of these terrorist soldiers being given sex slaves: kidnapped teenage (or younger) girls forced into sex slavery.

I'm sure a lot of these soldiers are 'press ganged' (forced) into these organisations against their will, but if they protest they will be tortured and/or killed. So these guys are scared as well, and are forced into committing atrocities.

Everybody needs to be educated about Islam. Many, if not most, Islamic leaders want to impose the religion of Islam on everyone on this planet. By force if necessary. Whatever it takes.

Here are two presentations by Bill Federer about Islam. I haven't seen the second one but the first one (The Rise of Islam) is excellent. You may have to copy and paste the link into your browser.

The Rise of Islam
www.youtube.com/watch?v=rKY4c4q33R4

The Real Truth of Islam
www.youtube.com/watch?v=LlNVfIuObS8

And many thanks Bill for your great courage in exposing the truths about Islam!

There are many good (and scared) Muslims and I am not opposed to them but I *am* opposed to the religion of Islam and to any Islamic extremist who wants to force his or her religion on me.
I like Zack's line: "Step back, I know who I am!".

———

Zack de la Rocha and Rage Against the Machine

If you are familiar with the band Rage Against the Machine you should have heard about two men in prison: A Native American activist called Leonard Peltier and a political activist called Mumia Abu-Jamal. Zack says that these men are innocent. If Zack says they are innocent I believe it. Let these men go.

There is a prophecy in 2 Thessalonians 2:3-4…

—Let no man deceive you by any means: for that day shall not come, except there come a falling away first, and that man of sin be revealed, the son of perdition; Who opposeth and exalteth himself above all that is called God, or that is worshipped; so that he as God sitteth in the temple of God, shewing himself that he is God.—

In some translations of the Bible "man of sin" is rendered "man of lawlessness". For years I pondered whether Zack de la Rocha was this "man of lawlessness". I loved Rage Against the Machine when I first heard them (in 1993) but in the nine years I was a Christian (2012-2021) I couldn't decide whether Zack was right or wrong. I heard him sing/rap the song "Fuck the Police". I think we need Law and Order, we need police. I wrote in earlier versions of this article that I thought that there were some bad cops, maybe a lot of them. But I have also met some police who I thought were the finest people I had ever met.

Bono sang: "it's no secret that our world is in darkness tonight". I see huge evil in the world. It seems to me that some unknown, invisible power or force is "taking over". Trying to subdue us, control us. To what end I don't know but for 27 years of my life something definitely was trying to control me, subdue me.

What's my point? Everyone needs a bit of Zack de la Rocha in them. Zack epitomises courage, fearlessness. We all need his courage to overcome our oppressors. I'm thinking of the regimes in Iran and North Korea. These oppressive governments need to be overthrown. And China's reputation is pretty bad as well.

I recommend RATM's first album which is simply called Rage Against the Machine. Listen to the tracks: "Wake Up" and "Killing in the Name of". All ten tracks are brilliant. I recommend that young people listen to this album. The later albums are good too but in my opinion the first album was the most powerful.

And before I close listen to the album 'Psalm 69' by Ministry. Listen to Al Jourgensen's pain. I know all about this type of pain. And how to overcome it.

UFOs and Alien Abductions

I have seen some films and documentaries about alien abductions. I read the famous book 'Communion', one man's account of his experience of alien abductions. And I have read about aliens removing foetus' from pregnant women for God only knows what evil purpose. Twice in my life I have seen lights in the sky moving very fast and zig-zagging in a way impossible for planes or helicopters. I have heard of a former Governor of Arizona state in the US describe seeing a very large spaceship. Here's a quote from the CNN website...

——Fife Symington says he nearly had a close encounter while governor of Arizona

(CNN) -- In 1997, during my second term as governor of Arizona, I saw something that defied logic and challenged my reality.

I witnessed a massive delta-shaped, craft silently navigate over Squaw Peak, a mountain range in Phoenix, Arizona. It was truly breathtaking. I was absolutely stunned because I was turning to the west looking for the distant Phoenix Lights.

To my astonishment this apparition appeared; this dramatically large, very distinctive leading edge with some enormous lights was travelling through the Arizona sky.

As a pilot and a former Air Force Officer, I can definitively say that this craft did not resemble any man-made object I'd ever seen. And it was certainly not high-altitude flares because flares don't fly in formation.

The incident was witnessed by hundreds -- if not thousands -- of people in Arizona, and my office was besieged with phone calls from very concerned Arizonians.

The growing hysteria intensified when the story broke nationally. I decided to lighten the mood of the state by calling a press conference where my chief of staff arrived in an alien costume. We managed to lessen the sense of panic but, at the same time, upset many of my constituents.

I would now like to set the record straight. I never meant to ridicule anyone. My office did make inquiries as to the origin of the craft, but to this day they remain unanswered.

Eventually the Air Force claimed responsibility stating that they dropped flares.

This is indicative of the attitude from official channels. We get explanations that fly in the face of the facts. Explanations like weather balloons, swamp gas and military flares.

I was never happy with the Air Force's silly explanation. There might very well have been military flares in the sky that evening, but what I and hundreds of others saw had nothing to do with that.

I now know that I am not alone. There are many high-ranking military, aviation and government officials who share my concerns. While on active duty, they have either witnessed a UFO incident or have conducted an official investigation into UFO cases relevant to aviation safety and national security.

By speaking out with me, these people are putting their reputations on the line. They have fought in wars, guarded top secret weapons arsenals and protected our nation's skies.

We want the government to stop putting out stories that perpetuate the myth that all UFOs can be explained away in down-to-earth conventional terms. Investigations need to be re-opened, documents need to be unsealed and the idea of an open dialogue can no longer be shunned.

Incidents like these are not going away. About a year ago, Chicago's O'Hare International Airport experienced a UFO event that made national and international headlines.

What I saw in the Arizona sky goes beyond conventional explanations. When it comes to events of this nature that are still completely unsolved, we deserve more openness in government, especially our own.——

And nobody wants to know! People don't want to think about such things and simply pretend to themselves that UFOs don't exist, that abductions do not occur. For them it's an SEP (an acronym coined by the writer Douglas Adams). SEP stands for Somebody Else's Problem. Most people couldn't care less about UFOs and aliens and abductions just so long as they themselves are not affected.

I'm deeply concerned about UFOs. Where do they come from? What do they want? Are they taking over the planet? And if so what can we do to fight back?

I have seen images of 'grays'. Tall thin humanoid creatures with large bald heads and all black eyes (no iris or white of the eye). It is absolutely clear to me that they are not natural creatures, they are the product of some sophisticated genetic engineering.

Perhaps they are genetically modified humans from our future (Earth's future). I read somewhere (possibly Stephen Hawking's A Brief History of Time) that there is some mathematics for time travel. That there are some theories on how it might be done. If time travel is, or will be a reality then the implications and the possible consequences are staggering.

Or maybe the 'grays' are from a different solar system. Either way they still look like genetically modified creatures to me. And up to no good I'll bet.

By the way, I am dead against genetically modifying *any* life form, from a beetle to a stalk of wheat to a cow to a human. It is unnatural and to me is an abomination.

Part 4 - begun 17th May 2022

A Design For Life

A shout out to The Manic Street Preachers for their song: A Design For Life.

Shit and Piss should not be pumped into our rivers and streams. They should be collected and used as fertiliser on the land. The more shit and piss pumped into our rivers and streams the greater the strain on the land's ability to sustain plant growth. Shit and Piss are like Gold to the soil and should not be squandered as sewage.

And what about poisonous chemicals and toxic waste that are poured into our rivers and streams? These should never have been produced in the first place.

We are poisoning and polluting our clean water supply more and more as time goes on.

When I was a child my Dad used to take me and my brother to "the bogs" which was the name for a small area of land at the edge of the Bandon river. We would all go swimming there. It was heaven. And it was free! Rich kids and poor kids alike all swam there. I loved going to the bogs. Some of my happiest memories are of swimming in the bogs as a child. I would drink some of the water as I swam.

But the water is polluted now. My father says that the river is too polluted to swim there now and we don't swim in the Bandon river any more.

———————

I read somewhere that a piece of land used for grazing beef cattle that could feed ten people for a year could feed a hundred people for a year if the land was used for growing vegetables instead.

———————

I believe that the raw Fruit and Nuts (exclusively) diet is not only viable, but it is the optimal diet. If the whole world was on this diet there would be no need for beef or dairy cattle farms and all the hard work that is associated with them. And as regards crops there would be no need to plough and sow fields every year.

What I'm thinking of is planting trees that yield fruit and planting trees that yield nuts on every piece of land that is available, including small pieces of land in towns and cities where other trees grow. Do you remember the short story about Johnny Appleseed? Young people probably aren't familiar with it. If you don't know the story look it up on the internet.

With this scenario very little work is involved. Once the trees grow they will produce food for years, perhaps a hundred years, perhaps a lot more than a hundred years. And the work involved would be a *lot* less than in conventional agriculture. Either pluck the fruit or nuts when they are nearly ripe (they will keep longer) or place a few nets around the trunks of the trees and collect the fruit and nuts when they are ripe and fall off the trees naturally.

I am 52 years old and as I write these words (May 2022) I feel like I am full of energy and vitality and I am currently just eating vegan food and drinking lots of water. I have a fair idea that if I upgraded my diet to just raw fruit and nuts exclusively my energy levels would go through the roof.

I just had my blood pressure checked. It was very high. I think that with my lifestyle it's meant to be high. It's not a sign of sickness but the opposite: a sign of well being.

I think that on a fruit and nut diet I might live as long as Methuselah (969 years). Perhaps I might even live forever! I'm not fooling here, I'm deadly serious, I mean what I say. I can feel it in my body.

A friend of mine raised the objection that on a fruit and nuts diet we would have nothing to eat over the winter or the off-season. Not so. Some fruits (e.g. apples) will keep for months if properly stored. And dried fruits (raisins, banana chips, dried apricots, sultanas, figs, dates and many more) will keep for a long time, perhaps a year, perhaps longer. And raw nuts will keep for months as well, if they are properly stored.

The Garden of Eden

Jim Carrey, what do you think of all this?

42

Chapter Two
Flesh

Is eating flesh good for you? Is it acceptable? Lions and tigers kill and eat grazing animals. So if they eat flesh why shouldn't we?
I read on the internet that around 14% of the population of the planet is vegetarian or vegan. Many meat eaters would never kill, slaughter and eat a cow or a bull or a pig or a lamb themselves but they are quite happy to let others do the dirty deed for them. If they had to choose between killing and butchering and eating an animal themselves or eating a vegetarian meal many, if not most of them, would choose the vegetarian meal. So if all meat eaters who have qualms about killing the animals that they eat copped on and went vegetarian, that 14% figure would increase significantly.

I have read in numerous sources that some foods acidify the body and other foods alkalise the body. Foods that acidify the body include meat, fish, sugar, some grains and processed foods. Foods that alkalise the body include fruit and vegetables. (Lemons taste very acidic but have an alkalising effect when digested.) It seems (and I believe it) that, in general, alkalising foods are good for you and acidifying foods are bad for you. Flesh foods acidify the body and this is one of the reasons why I don't eat flesh.

But the main reason I don't eat flesh is because the killing (and eating) of animals is an abomination to me.

At the time of writing I read on the internet that cashew nuts are acid forming. I eat lots of raw cashew nuts and I have no problems with them. So this may be one exception to the alkaline = good/acid = bad theory. Or maybe raw cashews are really alkalising and the article I read was mistaken.

I also don't eat shellfish or eggs. I consider these to be 'flesh foods' as well. If a food is not plant based (i.e. not vegan) I won't eat it with the exception of honey. If no bees are killed when honey is harvested then eating honey is fine by me.

The Protein Myth and B12

Many people believe that if you don't eat protein (i.e. flesh) you will lose weight and waste away. This is a myth. Proteins are built from amino acids. A diet with a variety of fruits and vegetables should provide all of the amino acids necessary to build proteins.

The 9 essential amino acids are: histidine, isoleucine, leucine, lysine, methionine, phenylalanine, threonine, tryptophan, and valine. The right combination of fruit and/or veg and/or nuts will provide all of the nine essential acids needed to build protein in the body. Search on the internet to find out which amino acids occur in which foods.

What about vitamin B12? It is said that vitamin B12 only occurs in flesh and dairy products. So where do vegans get their vitamin B12? A friend of mine has been a vegan for the last 27 years. He does not take B12 supplements and he is in good health. Harvey Diamond (co author of Fit For Life) suggests that the need to eat flesh or dairy products to obtain B12 is a myth. Read the last two pages of chapter nine (on protein) of Fit For Life.

As I said in chapter one, I find the sight of raw flesh to be disturbing and eating it is even more disturbing. I believe that abstaining from eating flesh is 'good for you'.

Chapter Three
Milk, Butter, Cheese, Cream and Yoghurt

I was a vegetarian (I ate plant and dairy food) for most of my my life. In that time I suffered from indigestion pretty much daily and would have to take some antacids regularly. In January or February 2021 (IIRC) I embarked on a vegan diet (no flesh or dairy products). I noticed after a few days that I no longer had indigestion, I didn't need to take antacids anymore. This was for me a vindication of the vegan diet.

As I said in chapter one I also began to smell better, I didn't need to shower as often. When I went to the toilet I noticed that my stools no longer had a foul smell. Sometimes I thought they had a pleasant fragrance (I'm not joking here). Another vindication of the diet.

The condition of my skin improved. When I brushed my teeth I noticed that I no longer had bleeding gums. More vindications of the vegan diet.

When I was a child our family doctor used to say: "cows milk is for calves". As I said in chapter one, the image of a man sucking at a cows teat is bordering on the perverse. Another reason I no longer consume dairy foods.

Because of the reasons outlined above I would go so far as to say that humans were not *designed* to consume flesh or dairy products. I think we would all be better off without flesh or dairy.

I'm very happy with my vegan lifestyle and I won't be going back.

Chapter Four
Food Combining and
Raw versus Cooked

When you eat flesh (a protein food) your stomach produces hydrochloric acid to digest it. Carbohydrates (e.g. bread, sugar, bananas) are properly digested in a more alkaline environment. It seems that combining flesh and carbohydrates in a meal is not a good idea as the acid and alkaline neutralise each other and the foods are not properly digested. So flesh (and proteins in general) should not be combined with carbohydrates in the same meal. Some foods (e.g. most vegetables) are neutral and can be combined with either proteins or carbohydrates. For more on this subject I recommend a book called Food Combining for Health by Doris Grant and Jean Joice.

I have a notion that if you can't eat a food in its raw state then perhaps you shouldn't eat it when it is cooked either. Potatoes are inedible when raw but cooked potatoes (e.g. french fries) are one of the most commonly eaten vegetables on the planet.

Lentils need to be cooked before they can be eaten (although sprouted lentils are edible raw). Grains of rice are inedible raw but edible when cooked. Like I said, I have a notion that if a food cannot be eaten in its raw state then perhaps it should not be eaten at all (either raw or cooked).

When foods are cooked beneficial enzymes, vitamins and other nutrients are destroyed. I have read/heard from numerous sources that you get much more bang for your buck when you eat various foods in their raw state. I know of no other creature on the planet (other than humans) that cooks its food. Cooking seems to be peculiar only to human beings.

I practised yoga in my early twenties and foods that are high in 'prana' are recommended. Prana means 'life force'. Raw fruits and nuts are full of 'life force'. Cooking greatly diminishes the 'life force' in foods. Fresh and raw fruit and nuts are alive. Cooked foods are dead.

I'm a big fan of juiced raw fruits but not juiced raw vegetables. I have heard several nutritionists praising raw broccoli juice and raw carrot juice but these vegetables, in their raw state, don't appeal to me. I prefer my vegetables cooked in spite of what I said above about raw vs cooked.

At the time of writing I regularly eat, and enjoy, lentil and vegetable based vegan dishes (cooked). But I am gearing myself slowly towards a diet of 100% raw foods: fruits and nuts and seeds in their raw state, dried fruits, and not much else.

I have some qualms about cooking live foods. Do potatoes or lentils experience pain when they are boiled? Who gives a shit? *I* give a shit! When I cook lentils I boil the water first before adding the lentils so that their suffering will be over as quickly as possible. This is another reason why I am leaning towards a 100% raw diet.

For more on this subject of raw versus cooked I recommend a book called Raw Energy by Leslie and Susannah Kenton.

Chapter Five
What Can Vegans Eat?

Fruit is best eaten on an empty stomach so breakfast time is the ideal time for eating fruit. Some fruits should not be combined. Acidic fruits (e.g. lemons) should not be consumed with starchy fruits (e.g. bananas). I said earlier that lemons are acidic to taste but they alkalise the body after digestion. Fresh fruit smoothies are popular among those in the know about natural nutrition.

For a more conventional breakfast regular toast spread with vegan margarine and regular jam is acceptable. Many breakfast cereals are suitable for vegans (before you add the milk). Recently I have been eating breakfast cereals with almond milk instead of cows milk and I find these satisfying.

Vegan yoghurts are available in some stores. I have tried one almond based yoghurt and another coconut based yoghurt and these were pleasant. They can be used with fruit to make a fruit salad with a yoghurt dressing.

What about snacks? I quote from chapter one... "Some nights I made sandwiches from slices of white bread spread with vegan margarine and tahini (I love tahini), mustard, lettuce and either tomato or avocado. I liked these sandwiches a lot. Sometimes I had a banana sandwich with honey." My favourite snack last thing at night is a few handfuls of raw cashew nuts.

What about dinner? Stir fried vegetables are nice. As are bean stews and curries. Tofu and tempeh are popular meat substitutes. Vegan pizzas are catching on. I have eaten some 'chicken nuggets' made with pea protein instead of chicken and I found one variety of these to be succulent and delicious.

For those with a sweet tooth there should be a selection of vegan chocolate bars in your local health food shop. As I said earlier, if no bees are killed in the harvesting of honey then honey is an acceptable food for me.

Whatever about the 'enjoyment factor' of a strict vegan diet, the physical and mental health benefits cannot be denied (from my own personal experience). Sometimes I feel I am a bit bored with my vegan diet but there is no way I'm going back to my old (pre vegan) regime. I can feel the health benefits in my body. My vegan diet makes me happy and is well worth sacrificing a few 'forbidden' pleasures.

The farther I go on my vegan journey the more I enjoy natural raw foods. The following comes to mind...

Fruit (bananas, strawberries, melons, grapefruits, blueberries, seedless grapes, avocados and tomatoes)

Nuts (cashews, pine nuts, pecans, walnuts, brazil nuts)

Seeds (sunflower seeds, pumpkin seeds and sesame seeds)

As time goes by I enjoy these foods (fruit and nuts in particular) more and more.

Chapter Six
Psychiatric Medication

I believe that most physical diseases (e.g. cancer, arthritis, multiple sclerosis, fibromyalgia, colitis, myalgic encephalomyelitis, asthma, eczema) can be prevented or treated, if not cured, through proper diet. Lots of fruit and veg and nuts and no flesh, dairy or junk foods. Based on my own experience I believe that mental illness also can be treated and even cured through proper diet.

I lived with constant fear for 27 years from 1994 to 2021. I took some action to fight my condition... In 2003 I quit recreational drugs (marijuana). In 2012 I quit smoking. Early in 2021 I embarked on a vegan diet. I took up jogging. I had been slowly reducing my dose of medication (clozaril) from 350mg daily down to 50mg between 2012 and April 2022 (a ten year period). Just a few weeks into my vegan diet (on 20th March 2021) I conquered my fear. I described all this in chapter one.

I was very happy (and without fear) from 20th March 2021 until the middle of May 2022. What happened in May 2022?

At that time (May 2022) I was hospitalised (against my will) and was forced (against my will) to take a higher dose of clozaril. Every few days my dose would be increased by 25mg. When I reached 125mg I had an extremely bad reaction to it. I spent about six hours in terror in my room. I was terrified and confused. I couldn't think clearly. I was extremely tired all the time and felt like I was about to faint every time I stood up. I had a compulsion to spit all the time. It seems to me that the constant spitting was my body's attempt to eliminate the poisons in clozaril from my body.

I now had a *new* fear: that I would be forced to take a high dose of clozaril for the rest of my life. That I would turn into a zombie (I have seen a few psychiatric patients that look, and move, like zombies). I have read that the body is the temple of the spirit. It seemed to me that I was doing my best to *sanctify* my body while I was being forced to take poisonous 'medicines' that would *defile* my body. The injustice of it!

On my super healthy vegan diet I expect to live to be at least 100, and still be in good shape (if I don't have to ingest poisonous medicines every day). If I am forced to stay on my current dose (250mg clozaril daily) I think I would be lucky to reach the age of seventy. I don't want to lose those thirty years. Murder!

In late July 2022 I wrote down how I felt on 250mg daily dose of clozaril…

I feel like I am carrying two heavy suitcases all the time.

I feel like I am going to faint every time I stand up.

I feel tired all the time.

My long term *and* short term memory are impaired.

I can't think clearly (confusion).

I find it hard to deal with people.

I sometimes lisp and spit when I speak.

I have blurred vision.

I drool a lot when I sleep.

Were it not for my vegan diet (which is high in fibre) I would be constipated.

I can't do any physical work.

Mental work (e.g. in an office) would be difficult for me as well.

EXCEPTION: from 7:30pm to midnight I feel okay, presumably

because the effect of the clozaril wears off by 7:30 pm.

Every day I have to wait patiently until the evening for the few hours of freedom I have from the side effects of clozaril.

I have to say that compared to other psychiatric drugs and doses, the side effects of 250mg clozaril daily are relatively mild. I had a hellish few months on the drugs modecate and depixol in the late nineties. The slow, steady, relentless torment and torture that I had to endure at that time were far worse than anything I am experiencing now or have ever experienced since.

It often occurred to me over the years that most, if not all, of the psychiatrists (and nurses) who treated me never once tried a dose themselves of the medications that they forced me to take. What better way to understand how a drug works than to try it yourself?

If I were a psychiatrist I would try a small dose of any medication I prescribe to get a feel for how it works. This would be far more enlightening than whatever literature the profit-driven chemical companies write about their 'medicines'.

I suspect that any doctor or nurse who tried a psychiatric drug themselves and found it to be extremely unpleasant would think twice about forcing a patient to take it.

If it were up to me every patient on the planet would have the right to refuse any medication of any kind if they think it is harming them. This should be a basic human right.

If someone hears voices in their heads I believe those voices are real and not imaginary. In other words it's not a hallucination, someone, or something, is affecting the person. If someone believes they are being watched and/or controlled then that is real as well, not imaginary. I used to hear tormenting clicks in my ears for many years which mysteriously stopped (pretty much) not long after I became a vegan. These clicks were not my imagination, they were real. I think that the whole world is being taken over by something, possibly aliens and/or their machines and computers (which were possibly the source of the tormenting clicks). Most people find that idea too disturbing to give it any consideration and they prefer not to think about it and to live in ignorance.

I think that, in general, a chemical imbalance in the brain is *not* the *cause* of mental illness, it is a *symptom* of it. The *cause* of the mental illness (e.g. smoking, alcohol abuse, recreational drugs abuse, criminal or evil behaviour, poor diet) needs to be addressed, not the symptom. If this is done the chemical imbalance should come good. So instead of prescribing a smoker some 'happy' tablets have him/her quit smoking instead. Two wrongs (smoking *and* tablets) don't make a right. You have to quit the smokes, then your brain will be healthier and you won't need the tablets.

I have found that when I drink a few beers for two consecutive nights I feel lousy the on third day but when I drink red wine I always feel fine the next day. So I quit drinking beer. Because of my healthy and pure vegan diet my body is a very sensitive instrument. I'm better able to 'feel' what is good for me and what isn't. And this applies to my medication as well as to wine or beer.

I drink red wine regularly. Some nights I have as many as four glasses of wine (a full 750ml bottle) over the space of a few hours (I'm a very slow drinker). This might seem excessive to you but for me it is completely harmless. I feel *much* more 'inebriated' after 150mg clozaril (my night time dose) than I do after a full bottle of red wine. I'm not exaggerating here, I mean it!

I'll say it again, every patient should have the right to refuse any medication if they feel it is harming them. This should be a basic human right. Most of the psychiatric medications I have taken over the years I found to be unpleasant, very often extremely unpleasant (torture). I deem these drugs I was forced to take to be *poisonous*. If I am forced to take them this is a rape and violation of my person.

Chapter Seven
The Diet

These five steps are the steps I took on my road to recovery...

1. If you smoke cigarettes give them up.
2. Eliminate flesh from your diet.
3. Eliminate dairy products from your diet.
4. Embark on a strict vegan diet.
5. Aim for a 100% raw (uncooked) diet (i.e. raw or dried fruits, raw nuts and seeds)

I am very suspicious of synthetic drugs (either medicinal or recreational) that do not occur in nature. I have used raw garlic as a natural antibiotic a few times with success and no side effects apart from the bitter taste.

Chapter Eight
Wine, Marijuana and
Magic Mushrooms.

I have written about how I enjoy red wine with no unpleasant 'side effects' but I can only speak for myself. I know when to stop, when I have had enough, and I am always satisfied. But it may not suit you, the reader.

I used to smoke marijuana on and off between the ages of 18 and 33. I think my time could have been better spent. I have no interest in smoking it now and, for me, the *buzz* is overrated.

Some of my friends smoke, and enjoy, pot and they have no problem with it. They have jobs and a 'normal life'. So what's good for them is bad for me.

Marijuana is a 'wonder plant' with many and varied uses. It is legal now in some countries and some states in the U.S. It is often used as an effective pain killer and has other medicinal and agricultural uses. It's not for me though and I don't miss it.

I said in My Manifesto that I am not interested in drugs anymore and I prefer to be clear. This was true at the time of writing it but if it was legal there is one drug that I would have no qualms about taking: Magic Mushrooms (specifically Psilocybe semilanceata AKA Liberty Caps). Mushrooms are technically a *fruit* of the mycelium, a plant in or on the soil.

There are a number of species of mushrooms that contain psilocybin. I speak here only about the Liberty Caps species.

I have taken *moderate* doses of Liberty Caps around 20 to 30 times in my life. I would describe the experiences as exquisite, clear and beautiful with no hangover or bad 'come down'. How could something so good be illegal?

Some people think that LSD and Magic Mushrooms are pretty much the same drug. Not so, they are *miles* apart. LSD is made in a lab, a synthetic drug. LSD is made from a substance found in a fungus (ergot) that grows on rye and this substance is poisonous in it's natural state. I have taken LSD roughly as many times as I have taken magic mushrooms. *Every* time I took LSD (no exceptions) I had a lousy, unpleasant 'come down' or hangover usually accompanied by an aching in my spine. It would usually take about 24 to 48 hours to recover, to feel 'normal' again. With Liberty Caps, on a moderate dose (I never tried a large dose), for me at least, there is no hangover or bad 'come down' whatsoever. You get all of the good and none of the bad.

LSD was probably the most significant cause (among others) of my 27 year career of schizophrenia. I consider LSD to be one of the most dangerous drugs on the planet. I consider liberty caps to be benign, even beneficial, when taken in moderate doses (for most people, some people with a delicate constitution might not be able to *handle* it).

A moderate dose for me is around 25 mushrooms (that may sound like a lot but the mushrooms are very small).

I never hallucinated on my moderate doses of Liberty Caps, I just felt pleasant, very pleasant indeed. And like I said, there is no unpleasant come down or hangover (for me at least).

I heard a story about a girl who took a HUGE dose of magic mushrooms and had a hellish experience. If I remember correctly she feared for her sanity and I think an ambulance was called.

So liberty caps are dangerous in large doses but this is true of other drugs as well. In my early twenties I once swallowed a large amount of hasheesh and had a hellish time for a few hours. And I have written about my recent night of terror in the mental hospital when my dose of clozaril was increased to 125mg.

I'm not suggesting that you, the reader, take magic mushrooms. Who knows, you might have a very bad reaction to them. You might lose your sanity. Or you might pick and consume a poisonous species that looks similar to liberty caps and die. I'm just saying that, in my opinion, for me (I won't speak for anyone else) they are benign and I have no problems with them. It has been 19 years since I have had any recreational drugs of any kind but if Liberty Caps were legalised tomorrow (they are legal in some places) I would give them another go.

I like Liberty Caps Magic Mushrooms.

AFTERWORD

I have written about mood altering substances: clozaril, beer, wine, marijuana and magic mushrooms. On the 25th or 26th of April, 2022 I had been on a fruit and nuts only diet for a few days (and don't forget I had been strictly vegan for over a year) and I remember eating a banana and I thought it was the most delicious thing I had ever eaten.

It occurred to me then that for any human that has completely detoxed and cleansed their bodies, that eating fruits (I'm not sure about nuts, yet) would have a drug-like effect. A 'high' if you will. So, for the purified person a banana will give you one kind of 'high'. An orange will give you another kind of 'high'. Grapes... and so on. So each fruit has a different 'buzz' associated with them but it seems to me that your body needs to be cleansed and detoxed, to appreciate the 'buzz' of each fruit. It took me ten months, on a strict vegan diet, to detoxify my body. I imagine it would take a lot longer for people who eat flesh and/or junk food.

Check out my book on The King James Bible...

Some Observations on the King James Bible
ISBN 978-1-8381219-7-6

I have written and published eight books about a new musical tuning I came up with in 2016 which is called Eagle 53. It took me 21 years to work it out. Like regular Western music it has twelve notes per octave but some notes are a bit higher than usual and others are lower. Eagle 53 has many advantages over regular tuning (Twelve Tone Equal Temperament). These books are all available on Amazon and some other online booksellers. If you are interested here are the details...

Eagle 53 My Ultimate Musical Tuning - ISBN 9780956649294

This book describes how I arrived at Eagle 53, the math and the rationale behind it.

John's Rules Music - ISBN 9781838121921

Rules for music composition in regular tuning, my Eagle 53 tuning, or any other alternative tuning.

The Eagle 53 Pianist - ISBN 9781838121907

Eagle 53 Jazz Chords - ISBN 9781838121914

The two books above are for players of pianos or keyboards tuned to Eagle 53.

The Eagle 53 Guitarist Lush Chords - ISBN 9781838121938

The Eagle 53 Guitarist Jazz Chords - ISBN 9781838121945

These two books above are for guitarists who have guitars fretted for Eagle 53.

The Arabian Scale in Eagle 53 - ISBN 9781838121952

This is for Eagle 53 guitarists or keyboard players. It lists 507 chords that, if I'm right, will all sound good played in *any* order.

Eagle 53 Beatless Lutes and 19EDO - ISBN 9781838121969

This is two short books rolled into one. Players of fretted and stringed instruments (e.g. guitar, banjo, ukulele, mandolin) might find book 1 interesting and people into math and tuning theory might find book 2 interesting. And some luthiers will be interested in both books.

Check out my website...

www.johnsmusic7.com

John O'Sullivan

Sláinte

6th September, 2022

Lightning Source UK Ltd.
Milton Keynes UK
UKHW020744150922
408910UK00009B/808

9 781838 121198